# Your Everyday Vegetarian Meals

## A Complete Collection of Amazing Vegetarian Recipes from Breakfast to Dinner

I0145920

America Best Recipes

## Table of Contents

**Breakfast**
**Vanilla Apple Cinnamon Breakfast Oats**
Prep time: 05 min Cooking Time: 05 min Serve: 2

Ingredients

½ cup oats

1 cup of water

1/8 teaspoon salt

½ chopped apple

1 teaspoon cinnamon

¼ teaspoon vanilla

1/8 cup honey

¼ cup coconut milk


Instructions

Add oats, water, coconut milk, salt, apple, cinnamon, honey and vanilla extract to Instant Pot and stir.

Close and lock lid and turn to —Manual‖ pressure. Select 5 minute cooking time.

When the timer goes off, do a natural pressure release for 8 minutes.

Open the lid and serve!

Nutrition Facts

Calories 175, Total Fat 1.4g, Saturated Fat 0.2g, Cholesterol 0mg , Sodium 154mg, Total Carbohydrate

40g, Dietary Fiber 4.1g , Total Sugars 23.5g , Protein 3g

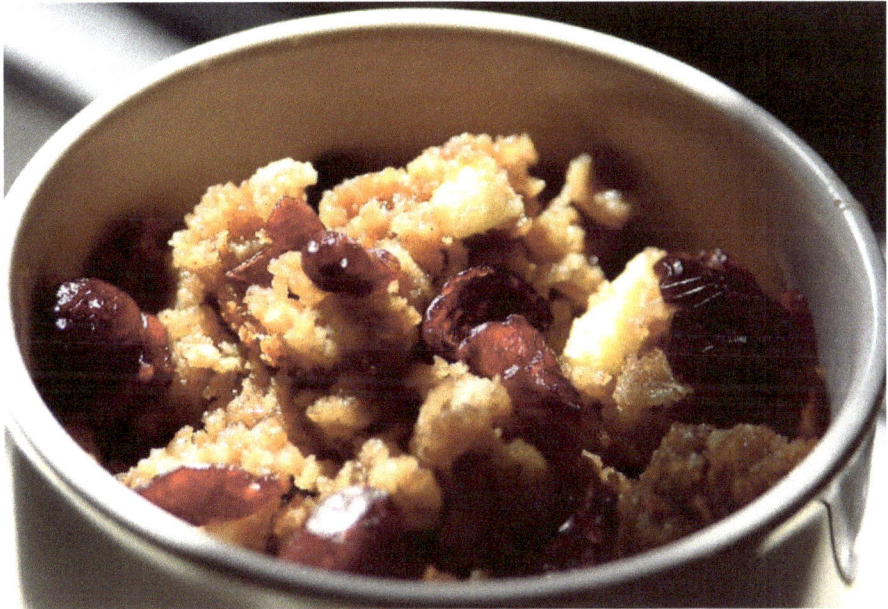

## Perfect Quinoa with Vegetable

Prep time: 10min Cooking Time: 05 min Serve: 2

Ingredients

1 teaspoon avocado oil

2 cups quinoa

2 -1/2 cups water or vegetable stock

½ cup broccoli

½ cup cauliflower

1 tomato

Salt and pepper

Instructions

Put the quinoa in a fine-mesh strainer and rinse under running water for a few minutes.

Press Sauté when hot, add in the avocado oil, vegetable stock and rinsed quinoa, cauliflower, broccoli tomato, salt and pepper.

Cover and lock lid. Make sure the valve is set to —Sealing‖. Set the Manual/Pressure Cooker button to 5 minutes on High Pressure.

When time is up, open the pressure cooker with the natural pressure release approximately 10 min.

Open the lid.

Fluff quinoa with a fork and serve.

Nutrition Facts

Calories 649, Total Fat 10.8g, Saturated Fat 1.3g, Cholesterol 0mg Sodium 33mg Total Carbohydrate113.3g, Dietary Fiber 13.6g Total Sugars 1.8g, Protein 25.5g

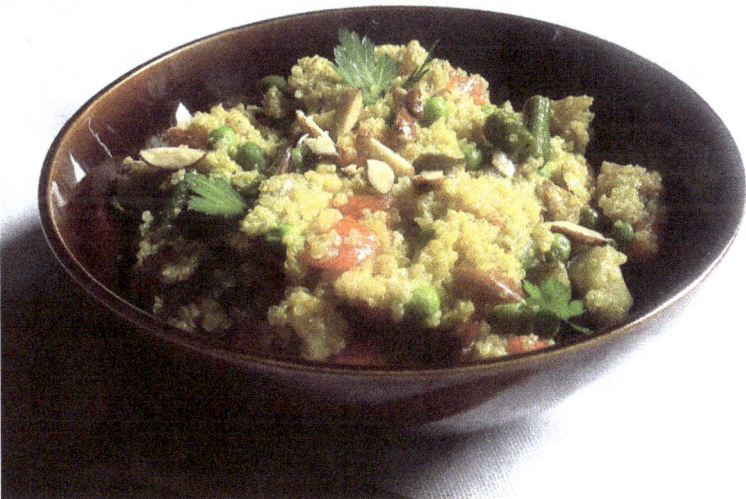

## Millet Vegetable Pilaf

Prep time: 10 min Cooking Time: 15 min Serve: 2

Ingredients

1/2 cup millet rinsed in a mesh sieve

1 tablespoon coconut oil

1 teaspoon mustard seeds

1/2 teaspoon dry ginger powder

1 small onion sliced thin

1 medium sweet potato cubed into 1/4 inch pieces (about 3/4 cup)

2 green chilies optional

3/4 teaspoon salt

3/4 teaspoon turmeric powder

1/2 teaspoon red chili powder

1 teaspoon coriander powder

1/2 cup peas

¼ cup tofu

2 cups water or vegetable stock

2 tablespoons chopped parsley

## Instructions

Slice onion, peel and cube sweet potatoes. Rinse the millet in a mesh sieve, it removes the bitter coating on the quinoa beads.

Turn Instant Pot on Sauté. When it's hot, add coconut oil and mustard seeds. When mustard start spluttering, add ginger powder, onions, green chili, cubed sweet potatoes. Sauté for 1 minute.

Add all dry spices, peas, tofu, millet, and vegetable stock. Stir well. Close lid. Set valve to ─Sealing‖ mode. Cook on Manual (High) for 10 minute. For a softer millet, cook for 2 minutes on the same setting.

Open lid after natural pressure release or quickly release after 5 minutes. Fluff the millet with a fork. Add chopped parsley. Stir with the fork and serve warm.

## Nutrition Facts

Calories 317, Total Fat 11.1g, Saturated Fat 6.6g, Cholesterol 0mg Sodium 895mg, Total Carbohydrate 44.8g, Dietary Fiber 7.3g Total Sugars 2.8g, Protein 10.7g

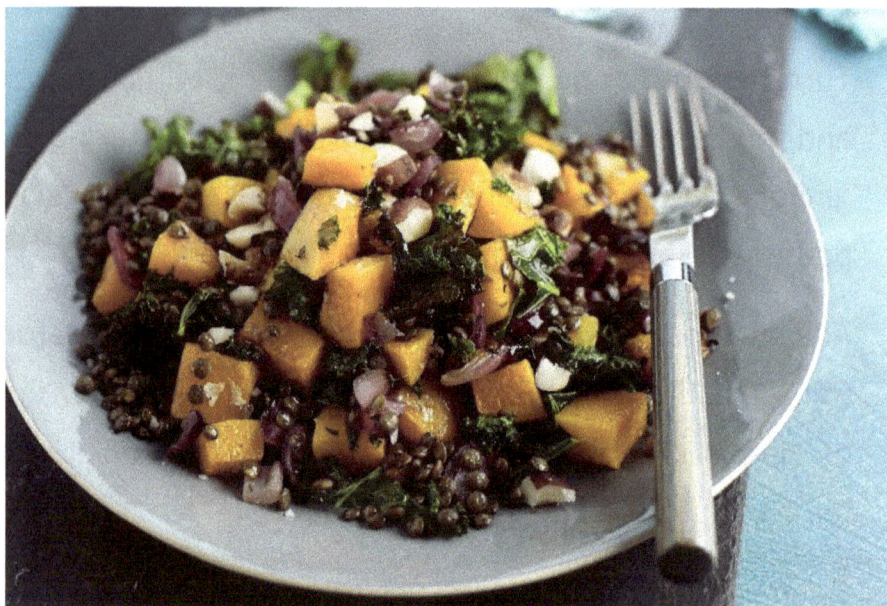

## Blueberry Banana Barley

Prep time: 05 min Cooking Time: 20 min Serve: 2

Ingredients

1 cup dry barley

2 cups water

2 ripe bananas

1 cup frozen blueberries for toppings

1 tablespoon honey

1 tablespoon chopped walnut

½ cup soy milk

Instructions

Place all ingredients in Instant Pot and cook for 15 minutes on High Pressure.

Manually release the pressure (Quick-release) when cooking is finished and enjoy.

Nutrition Facts

Calories 561, Total Fat 6.1g, Saturated Fat 0.8g, Cholesterol 0mg Sodium 52mg, Total Carbohydrate 117.9g, Dietary Fiber 21.4g , Total Sugars 33.5g, Protein 16.3g

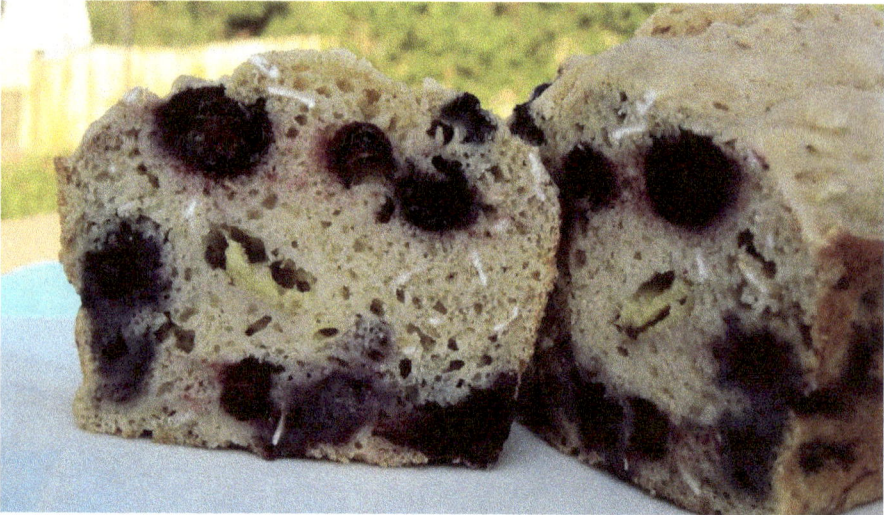

## Barley Pilau

Prep time: 10 min Cooking Time: 10 min Serve: 2

Ingredients

½ cup barley

2 cups water

1/8 cup raisins

1/8 cup shelled pistachios roughly chopped

½ lime zest and juice

2 tablespoons avocado oil

1/4 cup fresh basil chopped

Salt and pepper to taste


Instructions

Place the barley and water in the Instant Pot and lock lid. Using the Pressure Cooker function on High, set the timer for 10 minutes. Allow the pressure to release naturally.

Once the pressure has released, remove the lid. Add the remaining ingredients to the cooked barley.

Stir everything together to combine. Taste and adjust the seasonings, as needed. Enjoy!


Nutrition Facts

Calories 259, Total Fat 6.6g, Saturated Fat 1.1g, Cholesterol 0mg Sodium 47mg, Total Carbohydrate 45.3g, Dietary Fiber 10.2g, Total Sugars 6.8g, Protein 8.1g

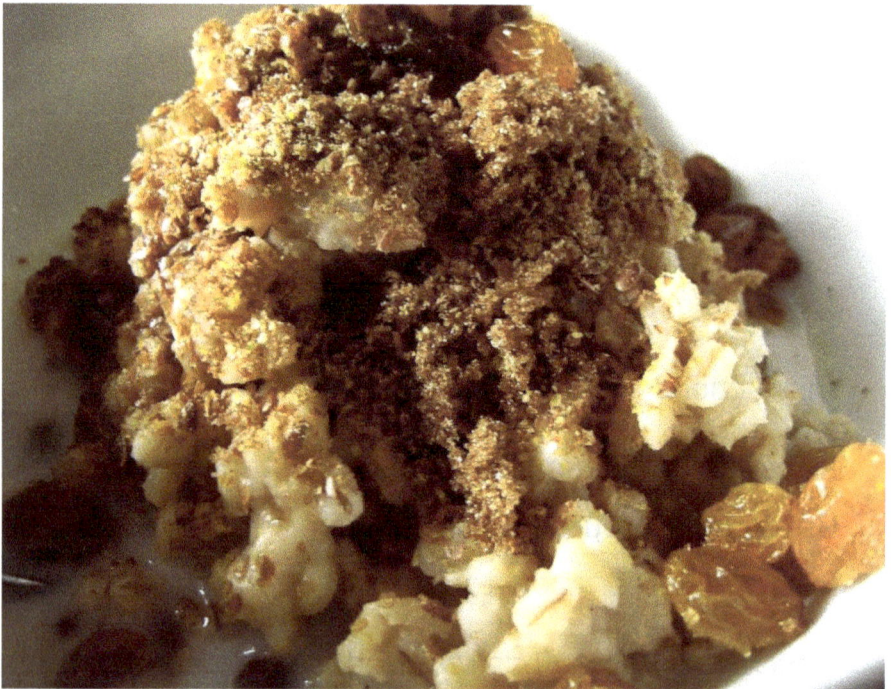

**Breakfast Cookies**

Preparation Time: 10 minutes Cooking time: 6 minutes

Makes 24-32

Ingredients

Dry Ingredients

½ teaspoon baking powder

2 cups rolled oats

½ teaspoon baking soda

Wet Ingredients

1 teaspoon pure vanilla extract

2 flax eggs

2 tablespoons ground flaxseed and around 6 tablespoons of water, mix and put aside for 15 minutes

2 tablespoons melted coconut oil

2 tablespoons pure maple syrup

½ cup natural creamy peanut butter 2 ripe bananas

Add-in Ingredients

½ cup finely chopped walnuts

½ cup raisins

Optional Topping

2 tablespoons chopped walnuts

2 tablespoons raisins

Directions:

Preheat the oven to 325 degrees F, and then use parchment paper to line a baking sheet and put aside. Add the bananas in a large bowl, and then use a fork to mash them until smooth. Add in the other wet Ingredients and mix until well incorporated. Add the dry Ingredients and then use a rubber spatula to stir and fold them into the dry Ingredients until mixed.

Stir in the walnuts and raisins. Scoop the cookie dough onto the prepared baking sheet making sure that you leave adequate space between the cookies. Bake in the preheated oven for around 12 minutes. Let the cookies cool on the baking sheet for around 10 minutes.

Lift the cookies carefully from the baking sheet onto a cooling rack to further cool. Store the cookies in an airtight container in the fridge or at room temperature for up to one week.

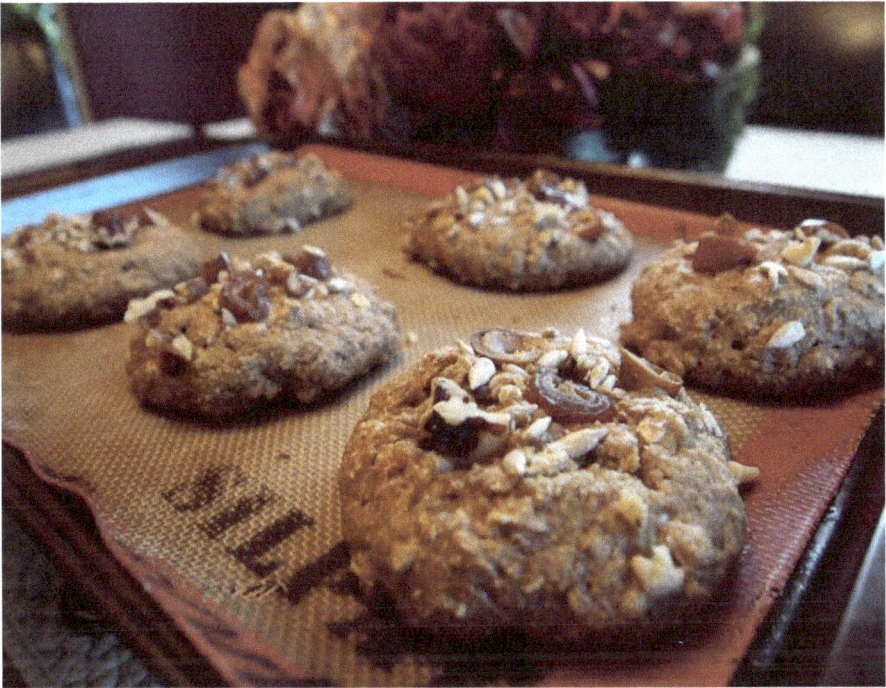

## Quick Breakfast Yogurt

Preparation Time: 2 minutes Cooking Time: 8 min Servings: 6

Ingredients:

4 cups Full-Fat Coconut Milk

2 tbsp Coconut Milk Powder

100 grams Strawberries, for serving


Directions:

Whisk together coconut milk and milk powder in a microwave safe bowl. Heat on high for 8-9 minutes.

Top with fresh strawberries and choice of sweetener to serve.

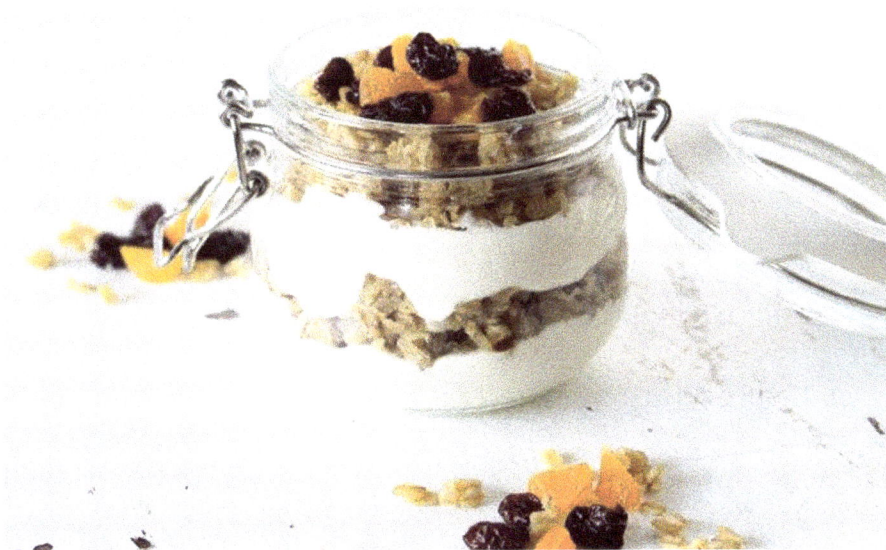

# Keto Breakfast Porridge

Preparation Time: 5 minutes Cooking Time: 5 minutes

Servings: 4

Ingredients:

1 cup Flaked Coconut ½ cup Hemp Seeds

1 tbsp Coconut Flour

1 cup Water

½ cup Coconut Cream

1 tbsp Ground Cinnamon

1 tbsp Erythritol


Directions:

Combine all ingredients in a pot.

Simmer for 5 minutes, stirring continuously.

## Scrambled Tofu

Preparation Time: 10 minutes Cooking time: 30 minutes

Servings: 4

Ingredients:

2 tablespoons coconut aminos

1 block firm tofu, cubed

1 teaspoon turmeric powder

2 tablespoons olive oil

½ teaspoon onion powder

½ teaspoon garlic powder

2 and ½ cup red potatoes, cubed

½ cup yellow onion, chopped

Salt and black pepper to the taste


Directions:

In a bowl, mix tofu with 1 tablespoon oil, salt, pepper, coconut aminos, garlic and onion powder, turmeric and onion and toss to coat.

In another bowl, mix potatoes with the rest of the oil, salt and pepper and toss.

Put potatoes in preheated air fryer at 350 degrees F and bake for 15 minutes, shaking them halfway.

Add tofu and the marinade and bake at 350 degrees F for 15 minutes. Divide between plates and serve. Enjoy!

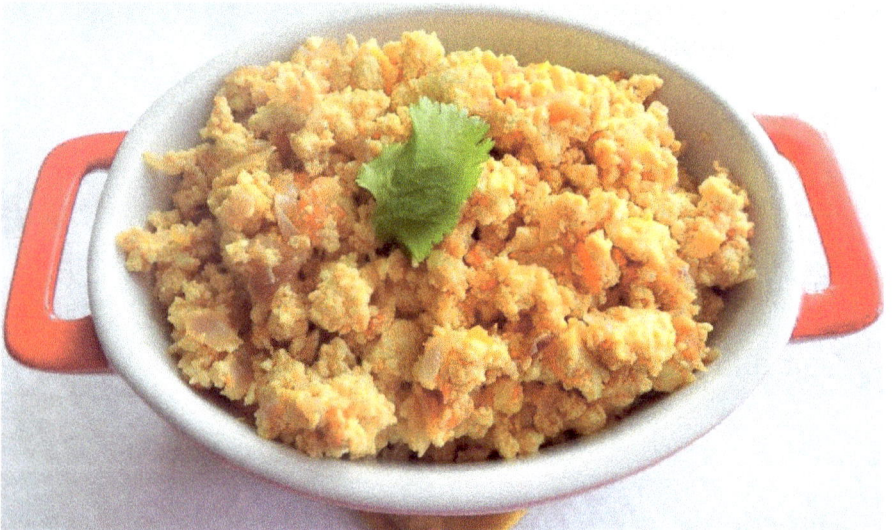

**Breakfast Polenta**

Preparation Time: 10 minutes Cooking time: 15 minutes

Servings: 4

Ingredients:

1 cup cornmeal

3 cups water

Cooking spray

1 tablespoon coconut oil Maple syrup for serving

Directions:

Put the water in a pot and heat up over medium heat. Add cornmeal, stir well and cook for 10 minutes. Add oil, stir again, cook for 2 minutes more, take off heat, leave aside to cool down, take spoon fools of polenta, shape balls and place them on a lined baking sheet.

Grease your air fryer basket with the cooking spray, place polenta balls inside and cook them for 16 minutes at 380 degrees F flipping them halfway.

Divide polenta balls between plates and serve them with some maple syrup on top. Enjoy!

**Lunch**

**Roasted      Butternut Squash      Bean Sprouts and Broccoli**

Ingredients

1 large broccoli, sliced

1 cup bean sprouts

1/2 butternut squash - peeled, seeded, and cut into 1-inch pieces

2 red onions, diced

2 large carrots, cut into 1 inch pieces

4 medium potatoes, cut into 1-inch pieces

3 tablespoons sesame oil

Seasoning ingredients

1 teaspoon sea salt

1/2 teaspoon ground black pepper

1 teaspoon onion powder

2 teaspoon garlic powder

1 teaspoon Sichuan peppercorns

Garnishing Ingredients

2 green onions, chopped (optional)

Directions:

Preheat your oven to 350 degrees F. Grease your baking pan. Combine the main ingredients on the prepared sheet pan. Drizzle with the oil and toss to coat. Combine the seasoning ingredients in a bowl. Sprinkle them over the vegetables on the pan and toss to coat with seasonings. Bake in the oven for 25 minutes. Stir frequently until vegetables are soft and lightly browned and chickpeas are crisp, for about 20 to 25 minutes more. Season with more salt and black pepper to taste, top with the green onion before serving.

# Roasted Brussel Sprouts and Broccoli

Ingredients

1 large broccoli, sliced

1 cup bean sprouts

1 red onion, diced

3 large kohlrabi, cut into 1 inch pieces

2 large carrots, cut into 1 inch pieces

3 medium potatoes, cut into 1-inch pieces

3 tablespoons extra virgin olive oil

Seasoning ingredients

1 teaspoon salt

1/2 teaspoon ground black pepper

1 teaspoon onion powder

2 teaspoon garlic powder

1 teaspoon ground fennel seeds

1 teaspoon dried rubbed sage

Garnishing Ingredients

2 green onions, chopped (optional)


Directions:

main ingredients on the prepared sheet pan. Drizzle with the oil and toss to coat. Combine the seasoning ingredients in a bowl Sprinkle them over the vegetables on the pan and toss to coat with seasonings. Bake in the oven for 25 minutes. Stir frequently until vegetables are soft and lightly browned and chickpeas are crisp, for about 20 to 25 minutes more. Season with more salt and black pepper to taste, top with the green onion before serving.

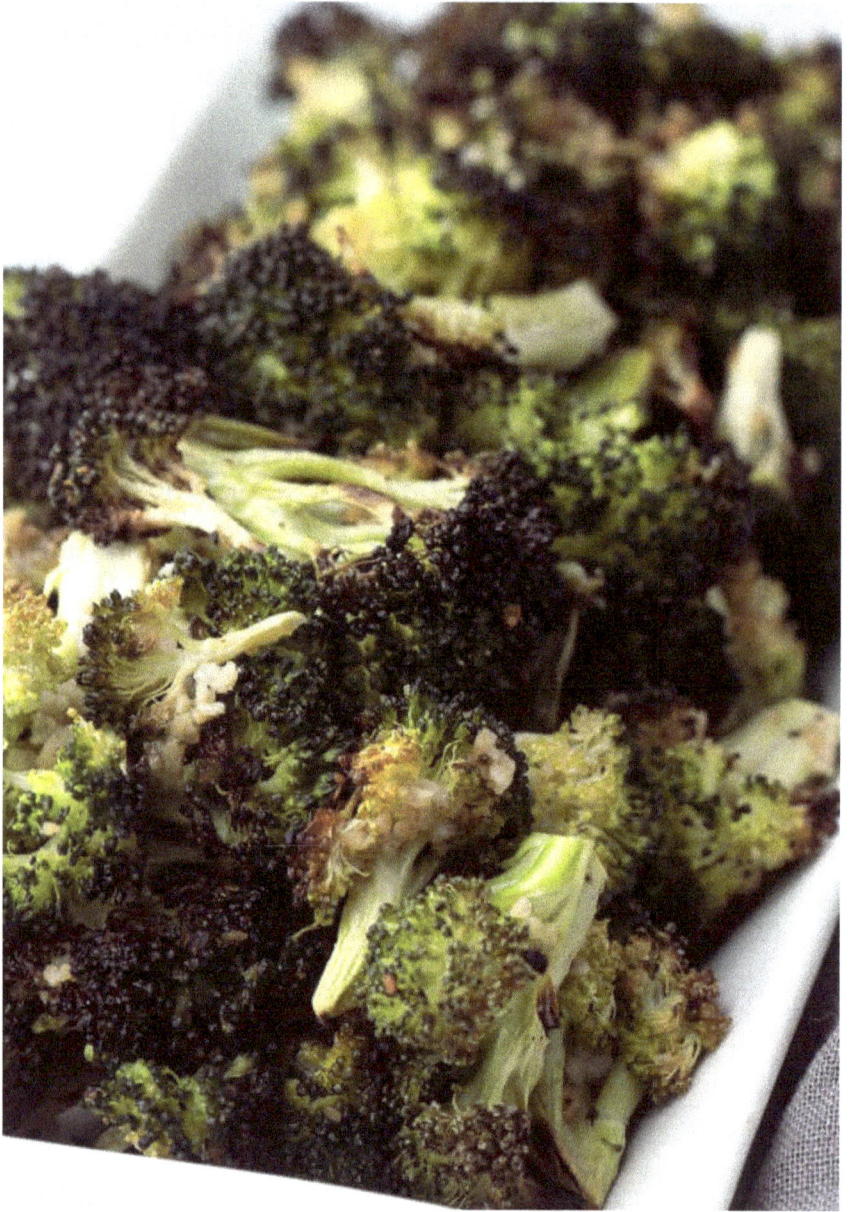

# Lemon Garlic Roasted Bean Sprouts and Cauliflower

Ingredients

1 large cauliflower, sliced

1 cup bean sprouts

1 red onion, diced

1 potato, peeled and cut into 1-inch cubes

2 large carrots, cut into 1 inch pieces

3 medium potatoes, cut into 1-inch pieces

3 tablespoons melted vegan butter/ margarine

Seasoning ingredients

1 teaspoon lemon salt

1/2 teaspoon ground black pepper

1 teaspoon onion powder

2 teaspoon garlic powder

Garnishing Ingredients

2 green onions, chopped (optional)

Directions:

Preheat your oven to 350 degrees F. Grease your baking pan. Combine the main ingredients on the prepared sheet pan. Drizzle with the oil and toss to coat. Combine the seasoning ingredients in a bowl Sprinkle them over the vegetables on the pan and toss to coat with seasonings. Bake in the oven for 25 minutes. Stir frequently until vegetables are soft and lightly browned and chickpeas are crisp, for about 20 to 25 minutes more. Season with more salt and black pepper to taste, top with the green onion before serving.

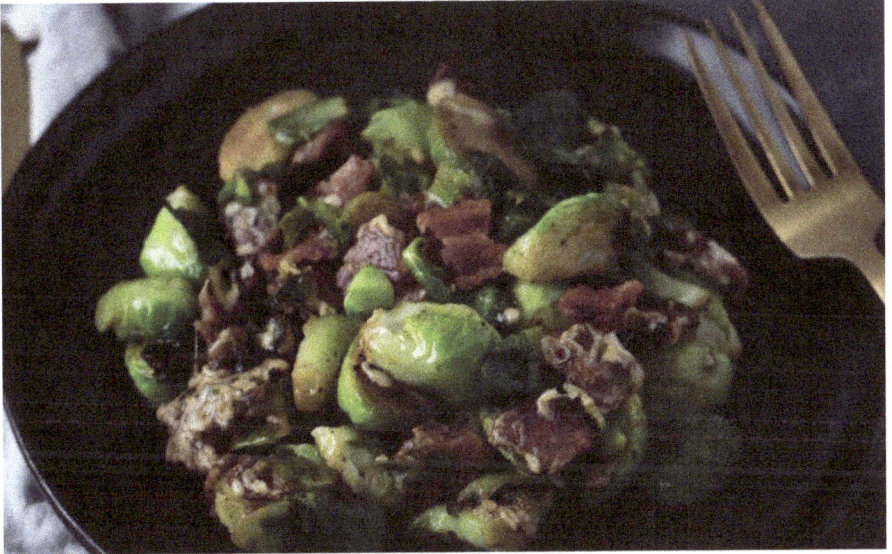

# Roasted Broccoli Sweet Potatoes & Bean Sprouts

Ingredients

1 large broccoli, sliced

1 cup bean sprouts

1 yellow onion, diced

1 sweet potato, peeled and cut into 1-inch cubes

2 large carrots, cut into 1 inch pieces

3 medium potatoes, cut into 1-inch pieces

3 tablespoons canola oil


Seasoning ingredients

1 teaspoon salt

1/2 teaspoon ground black pepper

1 teaspoon onion powder

2 teaspoon garlic powder

½ cup grated gouda cheese

¼ cup parmesan cheese

Garnishing Ingredients

2 green onions, chopped (optional)


Directions:

Combine the main ingredients on the prepared sheet pan. Drizzle with the oil and toss to coat. Combine the seasoning ingredients in a bowl. Sprinkle them over the vegetables on the pan and toss to coat with seasonings. Bake in the oven for 25 minutes. Stir frequently until vegetables are soft and lightly browned and chickpeas are crisp, for about 20 to 25 minutes more. Season with more salt and black pepper to taste, top with the green onion before serving.

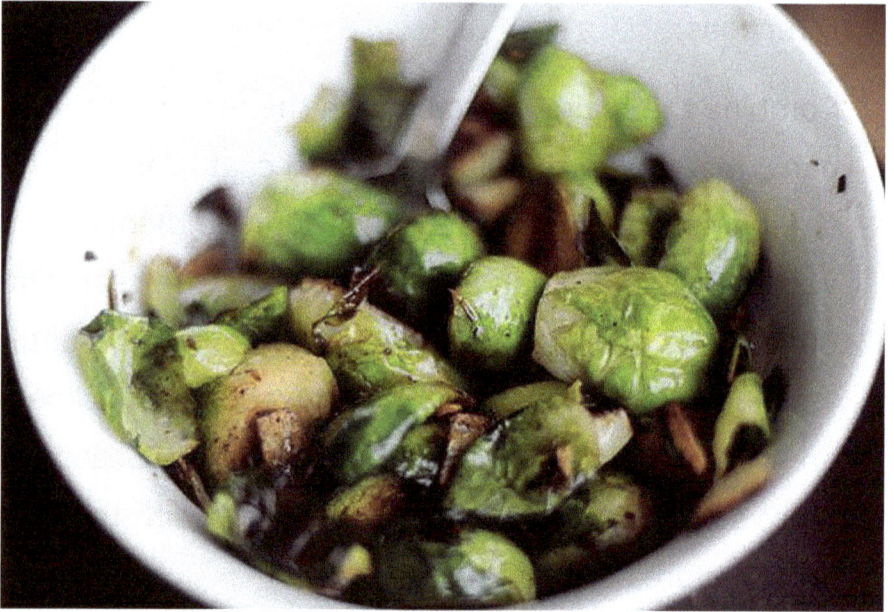

## Yellow Squash and Edamame Stir Fry

Prep time: 20 min Cooking Time: 10 min Serve: 2

Ingredients

1 tablespoon butter, or as needed

1teaspoon garlic powder

1 yellow squash, cut into bite-size cubes

1 zucchini, cut into bite-size cubes

1 green bell pepper, cut into bite-size cubes

1 cup edamame

1 tablespoon honey

3 tablespoons soy sauce

Salt and ground black pepper to taste

Enough water

Instructions

Select Sauté on the Instant Pot. When the pot is hot, add butter. Cook and stir garlic powder in fragrant for about 30 seconds. Add yellow squash and zucchini, green bell pepper, edamame, cook, and stir until vegetables soften about 7 minutes. Transfer yellow squash mixture to a bowl. Then add top with honey and soy sauce. 3-5 minutes. Add water, season with salt and black pepper.

Secure the lid on the pot. Close the pressure-release valve. Select Manual and set the pot at High Pressure for 5 minutes. At the end of the cooking time, allow the pot to sit undisturbed for 10 minutes, then release any remaining pressure.

Nutrition Facts

Calories 347, Total Fat 14.8g, Saturated Fat 4.7g, Cholesterol 15mg, Sodium 1385mg, Total Carbohydrate 33.4g, Dietary Fiber 7.6g, Total Sugars 14.1g, Protein 20.2g

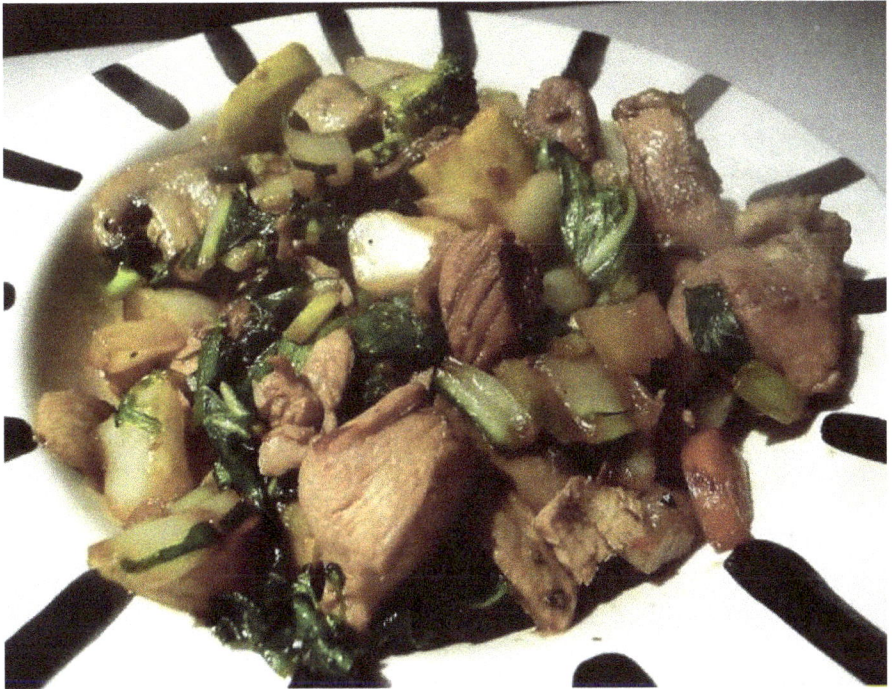

# Green Rice

Prep time: 10 min Cooking Time: 20 min  serve: 2

Ingredients

Oregano to taste

Few springs of coriander

½ cup mint

Salt and pepper to taste

1 tablespoon vegetable oil

1 cup vegetable stock

3 green onions

1 onion

1 teaspoon garlic paste

1 teaspoon cumin powder

½ cup green peas

1 green bell pepper

1 cup brown rice

Sunflower sprouts

½ green puree


## Instructions

Put the coriander, oregano, mint, salt and pepper, and 1 tablespoon vegetable oil, vegetable stock, and green onion in a blender and blend it well to make it into a puree. Select Sauté, add 1 tablespoon of vegetable oil to the Instant Pot, and add diced onions and garlic paste to it. Then add cumin powder, salt, and pepper. Mix them well. Add brown rice and pour some vegetable stock. Add green puree, green bell pepper, green peas, and sprouts. Toss it well. Lock the lid into place. Select Pressure Cook or Manual, and adjust the pressure to High and the time to 8 minutes. After cooking, quickly release the pressure. Serve hot.


## Nutrition Facts

Calories 607, Total Fat 18.3g, Saturated Fat 2.9g, Cholesterol 0mg, Sodium 146mg, Total Carbohydrate 95.6g, Dietary Fiber 10.9g, Total Sugars 8.4g, Protein 15.2g

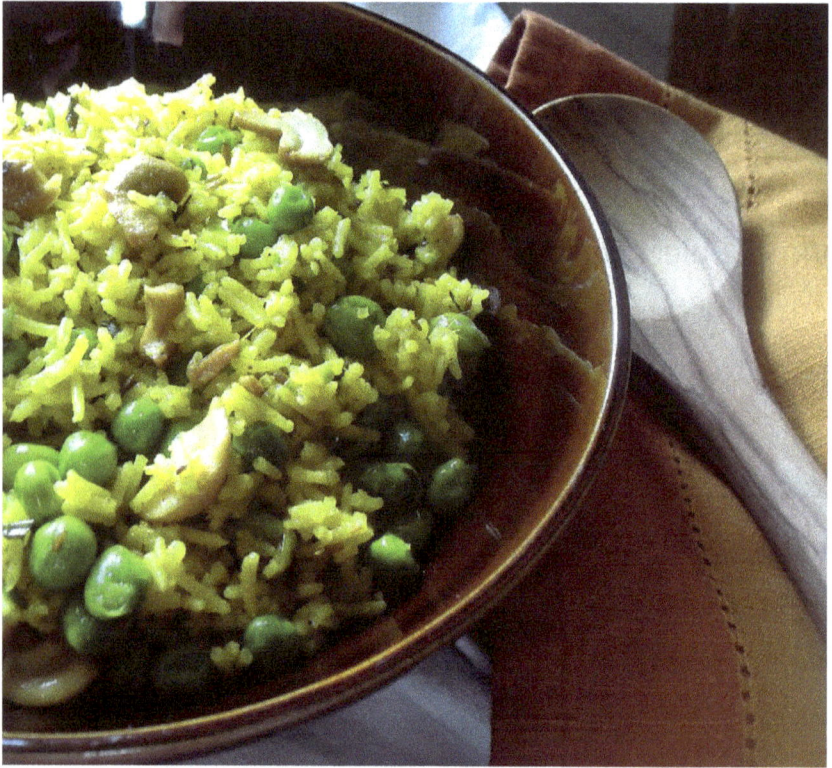

## Vegetable and Jackfruit Biryani

Prep time: 20 min Cooking Time: 30 min serve: 2

Ingredients

1 tablespoon coconut oil

1 small onion, thinly sliced

¼ teaspoon cumin seeds

1 whole green cardamom

1 clove

2 whole black pepper

1 bay leave

¼ cup carrots, chopped lengthwise

¼ cup green beans, chopped into 1-inch pieces

¼ cup white mushrooms halved

1/8 cup red pepper, chopped

1/4 cup green peas

¼ cup jackfruit, cubed

½ tablespoon ginger garlic paste

1/8 teaspoon turmeric

¼ teaspoon red chili powder

¼ teaspoon Garam masala

1 teaspoon salt, divided

¼ cup fresh coriander, chopped

½ cup long-grain basmati rice

1 1/2 cups vegetable broth

Instructions

Set Instant Pot to Sauté mode. Once the ─Hot‖ sign displays, add ½ tablespoon coconut oil and sliced onions. Cook for 5-7 mins until the onions are lightly caramelized.

Take half of the onions out and reserve for garnish.

Add remaining coconut oil, cumin seeds, cardamom, cloves, black pepper, and bay leaves. Cook for 30 seconds. Add all the veggies like carrots, green beans, mushrooms, red pepper, green peas, and jackfruit. Add ginger, garlic paste, turmeric, red chili powder, Garam masala, and salt. Mix well. Add coriander, rice, and salt. Add water. Mix well.

Close Instant Pot with pressure valve to Sealing. Cook on Manual for 6 mins. Quick-release. Open Instant Pot. Garnish with caramelized onions and coriander.

Enjoy hot!


Nutrition Facts

Calories 329, Total Fat 8.6g, Saturated Fat 6.3g, Cholesterol 0mg, Sodium 406mg, Total Carbohydrate

56.8g, Dietary Fiber 4.1g, Total Sugars 3.4g, Protein 7.9g

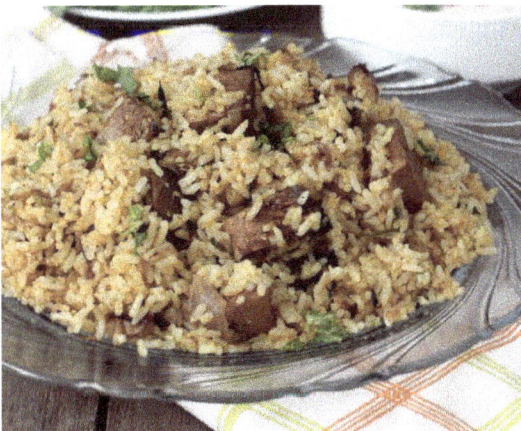

## Vegetable Millet

Prep time: 15 min Cooking Time: 10 min  serve: 2

Ingredients

1 cup millet, rinsed

½ cup mixed veggies like cauliflower, green peas, corn, carrot, and potato

¼ cup spinach, chopped

¼ teaspoon paprika

¼ teaspoon dried oregano

1/8 teaspoon ground cumin

1-4 pinches salt to your taste

2 teaspoons sesame seeds optional

2 cups water

Instructions

Rinse millet in water.

In the Instant Pot, add all the Ingredients mentioned above. Close and lock the lid of the Instant Pot. Make sure pressure release valve to Sealing.

Click Manual, then click Pressure, choose High Pressure. Set time to 10 minutes and walk away. It will take a few minutes for the pressure to build; after that, the timer will start.

After 10 minutes, you will hear the beep. Let the pressure release naturally for 5 minutes; after that, turn the pressure release valve to Venting. After the steam has ultimately released, open the lid.

A perfectly cooked millet is ready to be served. Serve mixed veg millet.

Nutrition Facts

Calories 404, Total Fat 6.1g, Saturated Fat 1g, Cholesterol 0mg, Sodium 26mg, Total Carbohydrate

75.3g, Dietary Fiber 9.1g, Total Sugars 0.3g, Protein 12g

# Beetroot Quinoa

Prep time: 5 min Cooking Time: 10 min serve: 2

Ingredients

½ cup quinoa

1 cup water

1 tablespoon coconut oil

¼ teaspoon cumin seeds

¼ tablespoon ginger powder

¼ tablespoon garlic powder

1 small onion, thinly sliced

½ beet cut into small pieces

¼ cup green peas

½ tablespoon lemon juice

1 teaspoon salt

¼ teaspoon red chili powder

¼ teaspoon Garam masala

½ teaspoon coriander powder

1/4 teaspoon turmeric powder

Instructions

Start the Instant Pot on Sauté mode and heat it. Add coconut oil, cumin seeds and sauté them for 30 seconds until the cumin seeds change color.

Add the sliced onion, ginger powder, garlic powder, turmeric powder, coriander powder, Garam masala, red chili powder, and sauté for 3 minutes. Add the beets, green peas, and spices. Mix well.

Add the quinoa and water to the pot. Stir the ingredients in the pot.

Change the Instant Pot setting to Manual and cook for 4 minutes at High Pressure.

When the Instant Pot beeps, do a 10-minute natural pressure release. This means let the pressure release naturally for 10 minutes, then release the remaining pressure manually.

Add the lemon juice and fluff the quinoa. Beet quinoa is ready. Enjoy homemade yogurt.

Nutrition Facts

Calories 265, Total Fat 9.8g, Saturated Fat 6.3g, Cholesterol 0mg, Sodium 1196mg, Total Carbohydrate

37.5g, Dietary Fiber 5.6g, Total Sugars 4.9g, Protein 8.2g

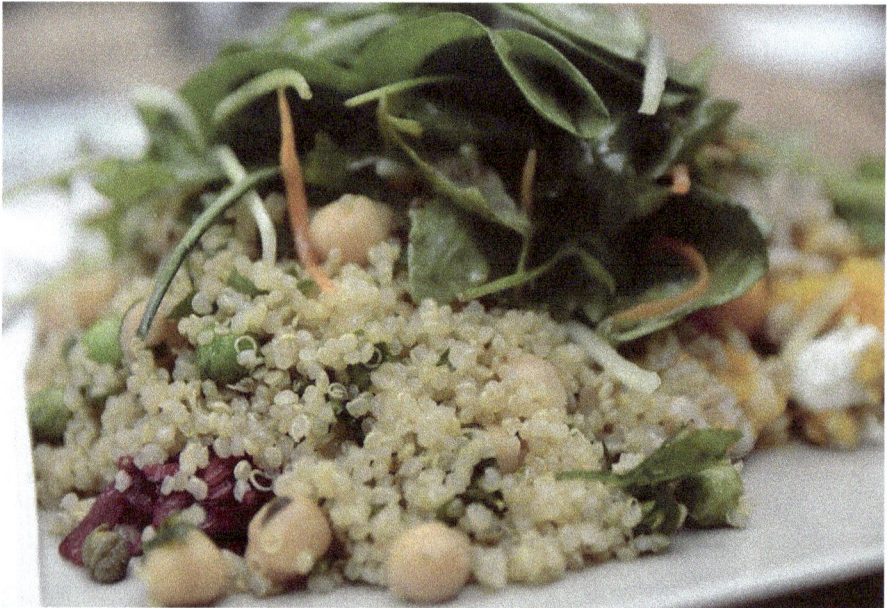

## Sun-Dried Tomato Risotto

Prep time: 15 min Cooking Time: 20 min  serve: 2

Ingredients

2 cups vegetable stock

2 cups sun-dried tomatoes, chopped

½ teaspoon garlic powder

1 small onion, chopped

Salt to taste

Freshly ground black pepper

1cup Arborio rice

1 tablespoon avocado oil

1/8 cup chopped fresh basil

Instructions

In an Instant Pot on Sauté mode and heat it, add sun-dried tomatoes with avocado oil, garlic powder, onions, salt, and pepper. Sauté for 2 minutes, stirring with a wooden spoon. Add the rice and stir for about 2 minutes. In the last 2 cups of stock and place, Stir change the Instant Pot setting to Manual and cook for 4 minutes at High Pressure.

When the Instant Pot beeps, do a 10-minute natural pressure release. This means let the pressure release naturally for 10 minutes, then release the remaining pressure manually.

Stir in cheese creamy. Garnish with basil and serve immediately.

Nutrition Facts

Calories 407, Total Fat 1.9g, Saturated Fat 0.3g, Cholesterol 0mg, Sodium 145mg, Total Carbohydrate 87.7g, Dietary Fiber 6.4g, Total Sugars 7.1g, Protein 8.9g

## Soups and Salads

## Summer Squash and Apple Soup

Ingredients

1 medium summer squash (1 lb of peeled and cubed butternut squash)

1 medium red onion, diced

2/3 lb carrots, peeled and cut into chunks

1 Fuji apple, peeled and sliced

3 cups vegetable broth

1 tsp. red curry powder

1 tsp sea salt

1 tsp black pepper

1/4 tsp cumin

½ can use coconut milk

Directions:

Combine the squash, onion, carrots, apple, broth, and curry powder in a slow cooker. Cover and cook on low for about 6 hours or until veggies are soft. Transfer these ingredients to a blender and blend until smooth Pour it back to the slow cooker, season with salt, pepper & cumin. Pour the coconut milk. Add more salt and pepper to taste.

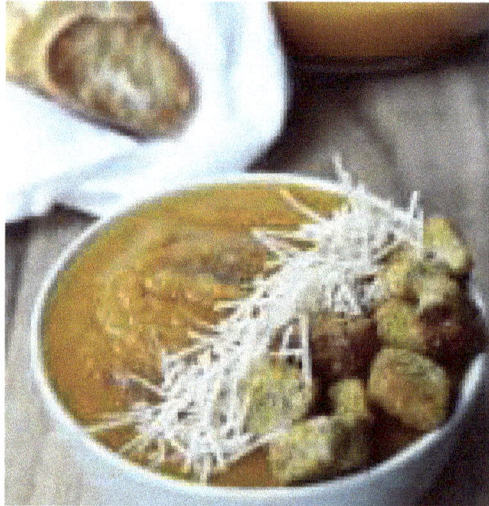

## Chinese Butternut Squash Soup

Ingredients

1 medium butternut squash (1 lb of peeled and cubed butternut squash)

1 medium red onion, diced

2/3 lb carrots, peeled and cut into chunks

1 pear, peeled and sliced

3 cups vegetable broth

2 tbsp. sesame seed oil

1 tsp sea salt

1 tsp Sichuan peppercorns

1/4 tsp dried ground sage

½ can almond milk

Directions:

Combine the squash, onion, carrots, pear & broth in a slow cooker. Cover and cook on low for about 6 hours or until veggies are soft. Take out the bay leaf and discard. Transfer these ingredients to a blender and blend until smooth Pour it back to the slow cooker, season with salt, pepper, sesame oil & Sichuan peppercorns. Pour the almond milk. Add more salt and pepper to taste.

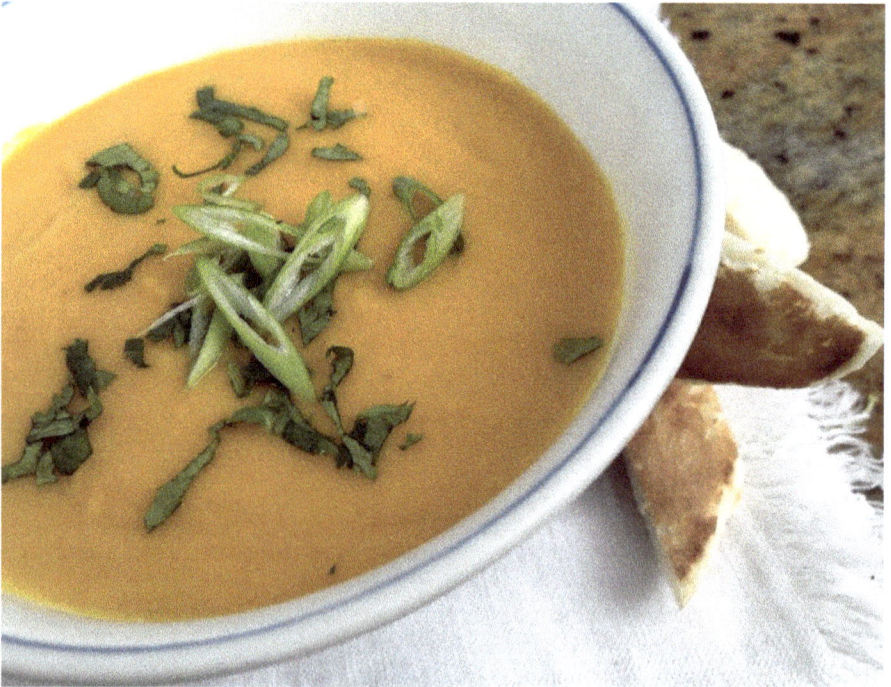

# Pinto Beans and Olives Tortilla Soup

Ingredients:

1 teaspoon extra-virgin olive oil

1/2 cup chopped red onions

6 cloves garlic, minced

1 cup vegetable broth

1 cup vegetable stock

1 cup salsa

1 14-ounce can pinto beans

5 pcs. black olives

5 pcs. capers

1 green bell pepper, chopped

1/2 teaspoon salt

1 avocado, chopped

1/2 cup loosely-packed cilantro

Optional: 1/2 cup crumbled corn tortilla chips Add olive oil to a pan and heat it to medium.

Directions:

Add onions and garlic to the saucepan and sauté until softened. Add the stock, salsa, bell peppers, capers, olives beans, and salt. Bring to a boil over high heat. Reduce to low and simmer for 5 minutes. Garnish with half of the avocado, cilantro, and tortilla chips.

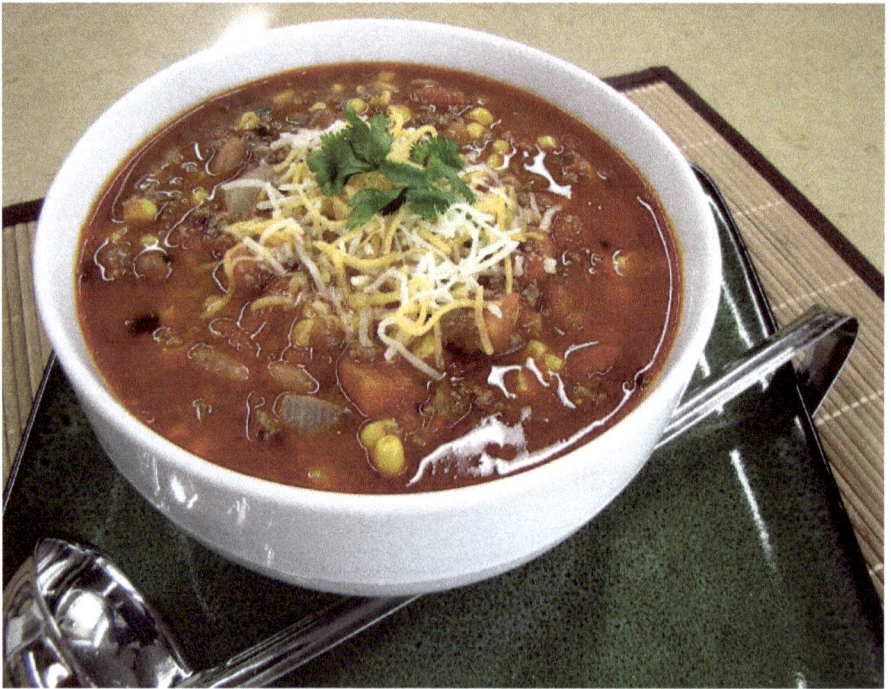

## Butterbean Taco Soup

Ingredients:

1 teaspoon extra-virgin olive oil

1/2 cup chopped red onions

8 cloves garlic, minced

1 lime, peeled

1 cup vegetable broth

1 cup vegetable stock

1 cup salsa

1 14-ounce can of butterbeans

1 green bell pepper, chopped

1/2 teaspoon salt

1 avocado, chopped

1/2 cup loosely-packed cilantro

Directions:

Add red onions and garlic to the saucepan and sauté
until softened. Add the stock, salsa, bell peppers,

beans, lime, and salt. Bring to a boil over high heat. Reduce to low and simmer for 5 minutes. Garnish with half of the avocado, cilantro, and tortilla chips. Remove the lime.

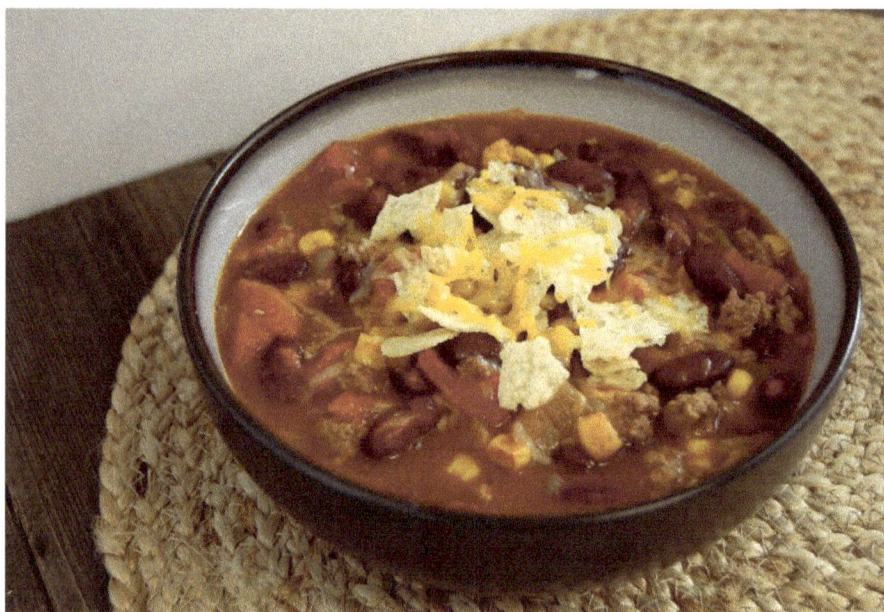

## Jalapeno and Soybean Taco Soup

Ingredients:

1 teaspoon olive oil

1/2 cup chopped red onions

10 cloves garlic, minced

1 cup vegetable broth

1 cup vegetable stock

1 cup salsa

1 14-ounce can eat soy beans

1 green bell pepper, chopped

1 Anaheim pepper, coarsely chopped

2 jalapeno peppers, coarsely chipped

1/2 teaspoon salt

1 avocado, chopped

1/2 cup loosely-packed cilantro

Directions:

Optional: 1/2 cup crumbled corn tortilla chips.

Add olive oil to a pan and heat it to medium.

Add red onions and garlic to the saucepan and sauté until softened.

Add the stock, salsa, bell peppers, Anaheim peppers, jalapeno, beans, and salt.

Bring to a boil over high heat. Reduce to low and simmer for 5 minutes.

Garnish with half of the avocado, cilantro, and tortilla chips.

# Asian chicken salad

Prep:10 mins Cook:10 mins Easy Serves 2

Ingredients

1 boneless, skinless chicken breast

1 tbsp fish sauce

zest and juice ½ lime (about 1 tbsp)

1 tsp caster sugar

100g bag mixed salad leaves

large handful coriander, roughly chopped

¼ red onion, thinly sliced

½ chili, deseeded and thinly sliced

¼ cucumber, halved lengthways, sliced

Directions:

1. Cover the chicken with cold water, bring to the boil, then cook for 10 mins. Remove from the pan and tear into shreds. Stir together the fish sauce, lime zest, juice, and sugar until sugar dissolves. 2Place the leaves

and coriander in a container, then top with the chicken, onion, chili, and cucumber. Place the dressing in a separate container and toss through the salad when ready to eat.

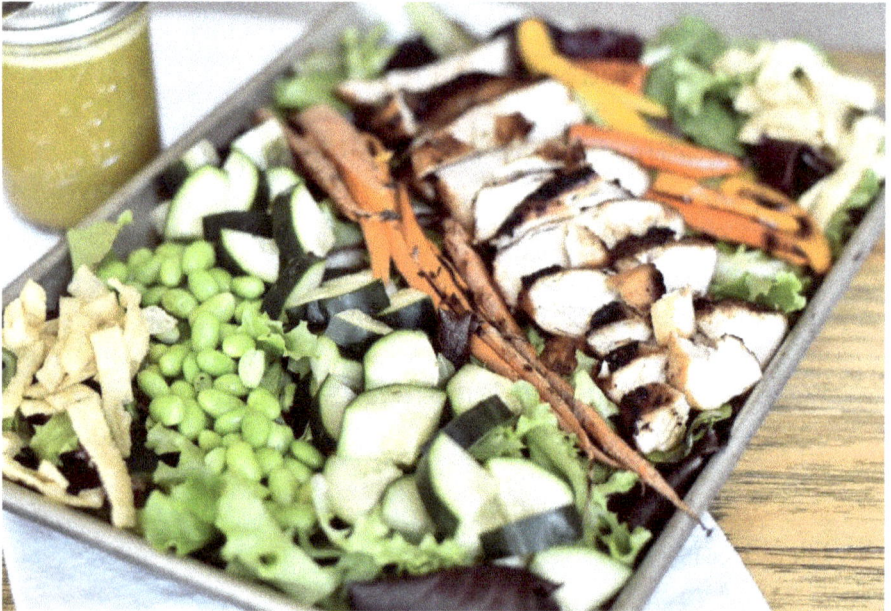

## Salad Tomato and Carrot Soup

Ingredients

2 tablespoons olive oil

1 small red onion, minced

1 small carrot, peeled and thinly sliced

2 large Salad tomatoes, thinly sliced

1/2 teaspoon minced ginger

2 sprigs of lemon grass

2 cups vegetable broth

2 tbsp. vinegar


Directions:

Sauté red onions until tender for about 5 minutes. Slowly add carrots; heat the oil over medium-high heat. Minced ginger, tomato, and lemon grass Cook for another 5 minutes, or until carrots become tender. Add vegetable broth and vinegar. Boil and simmer. Cook for 15 minutes longer.

## Kale and Quorn Pesto Salad

Ingredients

6 cups kale, finely chopped

15 oz. can borlotti beans, rinsed and drained

1 cup cooked Quorn*, chopped

1 cup grape tomatoes, sliced in half

1/2 cup pesto

One large lemon, cut into wedges


Directions:

Combine all of the ingredients in a bowl except for the pesto and lemon. Add the pesto and toss until coated.

## Lima Bean and Pea Salad

Ingredients

½ cup extra virgin olive oil

1 tbsp garam masala

2 (14 oz.) cans lima beans, drained and rinsed

½ pound ready-to-eat mixed grain pouch

½ pound frozen peas

2 lemons, zested and juiced

1 large pack parsley, leaves roughly chopped

1 large mint leaves, roughly chopped Half pound radishes, roughly chopped

1 cucumber, chopped pomegranate seeds, to serve

Directions:

Preheat your oven to 392 degrees F. Add ¼ cup oil with the garam masala and add some salt. Combine this with the chickpeas in a large roasting pan, then cook for 15 mins. or until crisp. Add the mixed grains, peas, and lemon zest. Stir and return to the oven for about 10 mins. Toss with the herbs, radishes, cucumber, remaining oil, and lemon juice. Season with more salt and garnish with the pomegranate seeds.

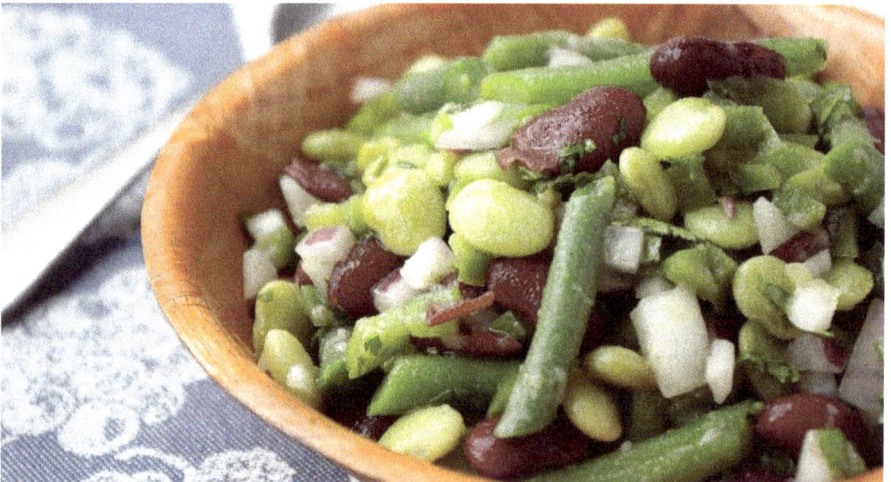

## Blueberry and Kale Citrus Salad

Ingredients

1 bunch kale, stemmed and torn to bite-sized pieces

1 lb. blueberries, sliced

1/4 cup sliced almonds Dressing Ingredients Juice of

1 lemon 3 Tbsp. extra virgin olive oil

1 Tbsp. honey 1/8 tsp. sea salt

1/8 tsp. white pepper

3-4  Tbsp. orange juice In a bowl, combine the kale, strawberries, and almonds.

Directions:

Combine all of the dressing ingredients and pour over the salad. Makes 3 to 4 servings

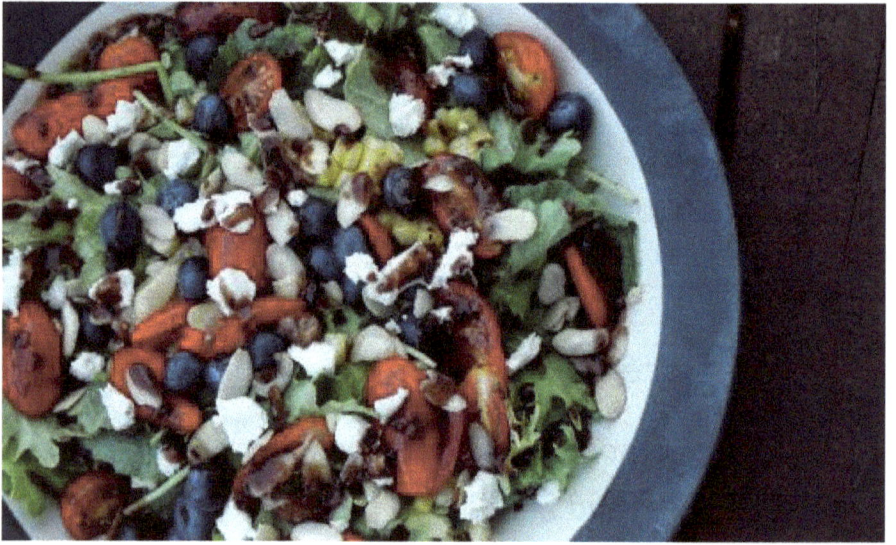

**Dinner**

**Shakshuka**

Prep Time 10 minutes Cook Time 10 minutes Servings: 1

Ingredients

1 cup marinara sauce 1 chili pepper

4 eggs

1 oz feta cheese

1/8 tsp cumin salt pepper fresh basil

Instructions

Preheat the oven to 400°F.

Heat a small skillet on a medium flame with a cup of marinara sauce and some chopped chili pepper. Let the chili pepper cook for about 5 minutes in the sauce.

Crack and gently lower your eggs into the marinara sauce. Crack eggs

Sprinkle feta cheese all over the eggs and season with salt, pepper and cumin.

Sprinkle with feta

Using an oven mitt, place the skillet into your oven and bake for about 10 minutes. Now the skillet should be hot enough to continue cooking the food in the oven instead of heating itself up first.

Once the eggs are cooked, but still runny, take the skillet out with an oven mitt. Chop some fresh basil and sprinkle over the shakshuka. Enjoy straight out of the skillet but be careful- it will remain hot for some time! Enjoy!

Nutrition Info

490 Calories 34g of Fat 35g of Protein

4g of Net Carbs

# Cheesy Thyme Waffles

Servings 4 total waffles

Ingredients

½ large head cauliflower, riced

1      cup finely shredded mozzarella cheese 1 cup packed collard greens

1/3 cup Parmesan cheese 2 large eggs

2      stalks green onion

1      tablespoon sesame seed 1 tablespoon olive oil

2      teaspoons fresh chopped thyme 1 teaspoon garlic powder

½ teaspoon ground black pepper

½ teaspoon salt

Instructions

Prep your cauliflower, spring onion, and thyme by cutting the cauliflower into florets, slicing the spring onion into small slices, and ripping the thyme off of the stems.

In a food processor, rice the cauliflower by pulsing it until a crumbly texture is formed.

Add the spring onion, thyme, and collard greens to the mixture and continue pulsing until everything is well combined.

Scoop the mixture out into a large mixing bowl.

Add the 1 Cup Mozzerella Cheese, 1/3 Cup Parmesan Cheese, 2 Large Eggs, 1 Tbsp. Sesame Seed, 1 Tbsp. Olive Oil, 1 tsp. Garlic Powder, 1/2 tsp. Black Pepper, and 1/2 tsp. Salt.

Mix everything together well until a loose batter is formed. Heat your waffle iron until it's ready to go, then spoon mixture onto waffle iron evenly.

Let the waffle cook as per manufacturers instructions. Remove from waffle iron and serve hot!

Nutrition Info

203.25 Calories 15.38g Fats 5.86g Net Carbs 14.99g Protein.

# Baked Eggs and Asparagus with Parmesan

If you like baked eggs and asparagus, you'll love this combination of Baked Eggs with Asparagus and Parmesan for an easy breakfast.

Prep Time 7 minutes Cook Time 18 minutes Total Time 25 minutes Servings 2 servings

Ingredients

8 thick asparagus spears, cut on the diagonal into bite-sized pieces

4 eggs, room temperature 2 tsp. olive oil

salt and fresh-ground black pepper to taste 2 T Parmesan cheese

Instructions

Preheat the oven to 400F/200C and spray two gratin dishes with non-stick spray or olive oil.

Break each egg into a small dish and let eggs come to room temperature while you roast the asparagus.

(Starting with the eggs at room temperature is VERY important.)

Cut off the few inches of tough woody part at the bottom of each asparagus spear and discard. Cut the rest of each piece of asparagus on the diagonal into short pieces slightly less than 2 inches long.

Put half the asparagus pieces into each gratin dish and put dishes into the oven to roast the asparagus, setting a timer for 10 minutes.

When the timer goes off after ten minutes, remove gratin dishes from the oven one at a time and carefully slide two eggs over the asparagus in each dish. Put back in the oven and set the timer for 5 minutes.

After 5 minutes (or when the egg white is starting to barely look set), remove gratin dishes one at a time again and sprinkle each with a tablespoon of coarsely-grated Parmesan.

Put dishes back in the oven and cook 3 minutes, or until the white is set, the cheese is slightly melted, and the yolk is still soft then you touch it with your finger.

Serve hot. I thought this was delicious just as it is in the photo, and loved the runny yolk on the pieces of asparagus, but you could eat with toast to dip into the egg if you prefer.

Nutrition Info

Calories: 217

Total Fat: 16g Saturated Fat: 5g Unsaturated Fat: 10g Cholesterol: 376mg Sodium: 530mg Carbohydrates: 4g Fiber: 1g

Sugar: 1g Protein: 15g

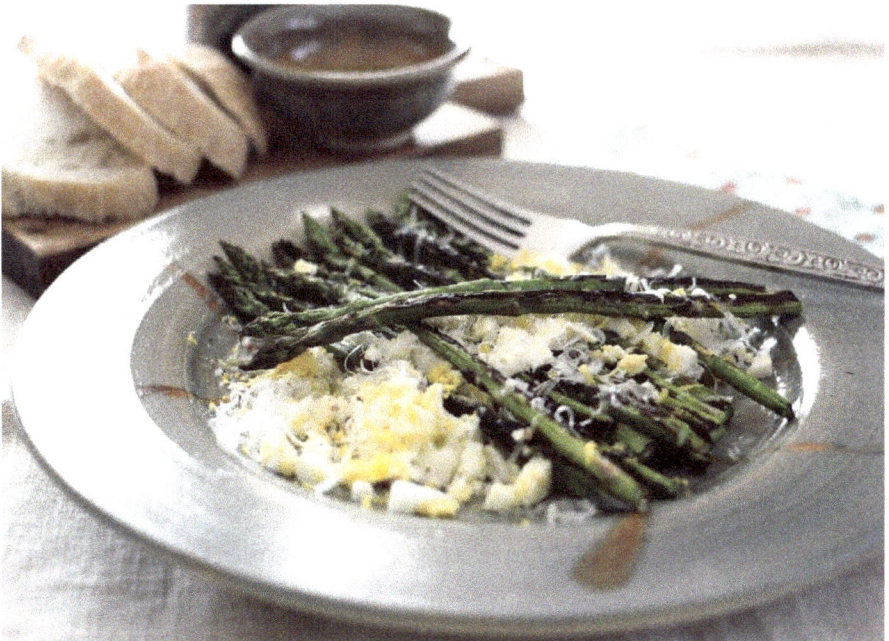

## Caprese grilled eggplant roll ups

These caprese eggplant roll ups are easy to make and make a great appetizer or snack.

Prep Time 5 mins Cook Time 8 mins Total Time 13 mins

Servings: 8 bites, approx

Ingredients

1 eggplant aubergine, small/medium

4 oz mozzarella 115g, approx

1 tomato large

2 basil leaves or a little more as needed good quality olive oil

Instructions

Make sure your knife is sharp before starting. Cut the end off the eggplant then cut it int thin slices, around 0.1in/0.25cm thick lengthwise. Discard the smaller pieces that are mainly skin and not as long from either side.

Slice the mozzarella and tomato very thinly as well. Shred the basil leaves thinly. Warm a griddle pan and lightly brush the eggplant slices with olive oil. Alternatively, drizzle on a little and quickly rub over before it is absorbed. Place the eggplant slices on the pan and grill for a couple minutes each side . They should soften and have light grill marks. As the second side is almost done, add a larger piece of mozzarella in the thick part of the eggplant slice. Top it with a slice of tomato, and add a smaller piece of mozzarella at the thiner end. Sprinkle over a couple pieces of basil and drizzle a little olive oil and a couple grinds of black pepper, if you like. Let it cook fir a minute more then carefully remove from the pan. There will be a bit of liquid comes out from the tomato and cheese so let it drain off. Roll the eggplant from the thiner end, which has only the cheese. You probably won't get it to roll completely, but once it's close, hold together with a cocktail stick.

Nutrition Info: Calories: 59kcal Carbohydrates: 4g Protein: 3g Fat: 3g Saturated Fat: 1g Cholesterol: 11mg Sodium: 90mg Potassium: 178mg Fiber: 1g Sugar: 2g

## Kale with Sweet Potatoes

(Prep time: 10 min |Cooking Time: 15 min | serve: 2)

Ingredients

2 cups kale, washed and chopped

2 sweet potatoes, washed and cut large pieces

1 cup water

1 tablespoon coconut oil

1 lime juiced, plus extra slices for serving

1tablespoon garlic powder

¼ teaspoon salt

1/8 teaspoon pepper

Instructions

Wash the kale and sweet potatoes well and chop.

Add everything to the Instant Pot and stir very well.

Cover the Instant Pot and lock it in. Make sure the vent is set to ─Sealing‖.

Use the Manual or Pressure Cook feature and set the timer for 15 minutes.

Once the timer reaches zero, quickly release the pressure. Enjoy!

Nutrition Facts

Calories 190, Total Fat 6.8g, Saturated Fat 5.9g, Cholesterol 0mg, Sodium 347mg, Total Carbohydrate

28.5g, Dietary Fiber 3.6g, Total Sugars 4.9g, Protein 3.8g

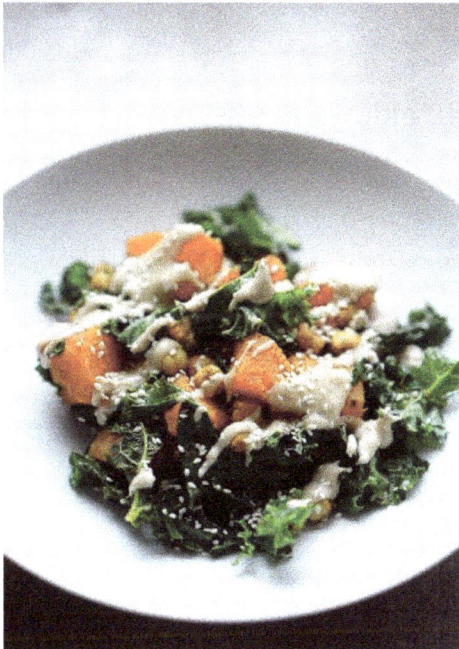

## Grilled Beetroots and Artichoke Hearts

Ingredients

1 cup artichoke hearts

2 beetroots, peeled and sliced lengthwise

1 large red onion, cut into 1/2 inch thick rounds

1/3 cup Italian parsley or basil, finely chopped

Dressing:

6 tbsp. extra virgin olive oil

Sea salt, to taste

3 tbsp. apple cider vinegar

1 tbsp. honey


Directions:

Egg-free mayonnaise Combine all of the dressing ingredients thoroughly. Preheat your grill to low heat and grease the grates. Layer the vegetable grill for 12 minutes per side until tender, flipping once. Brush with the marinade/ dressing ingredients

## Grilled Cabbage and Collard Greens

Ingredients

1 medium Cabbage sliced

1 bunch of collard greens

1 large red onion, cut into 1/2 inch thick rounds

1/3 cup Italian parsley or basil, finely chopped

Dressing Ingredients

6 tbsp. olive oil

1 tsp. garlic powder

1 tsp. onion powder

Sea salt, to taste

3 tbsp. white wine vinegar

English mustard

Directions:

Combine all of the dressing ingredients thoroughly.
Preheat your grill to low heat and grease the grates.
Layer the vegetable grill for 12 minutes per side until

tender, flipping once. Brush with the marinade/
dressing ingredients

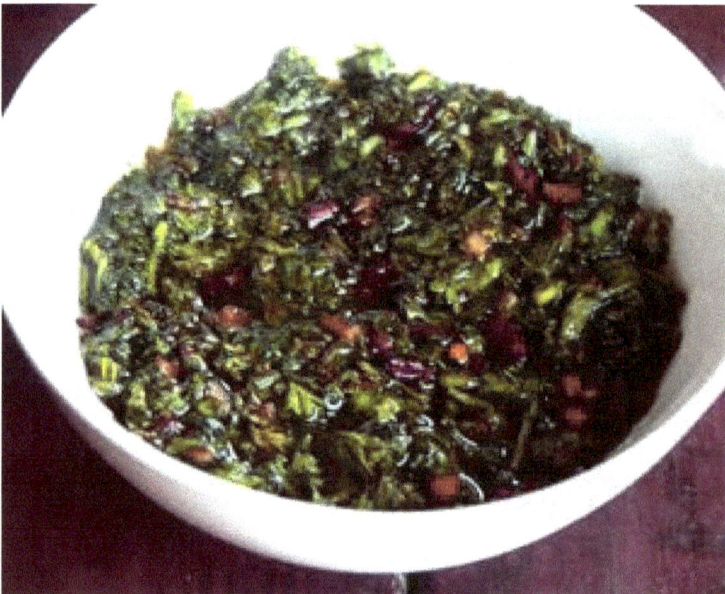

## Grilled Artichoke and Mustard Greens

Ingredients

1 pc. Artichoke

1 bunch of mustard greens

2 medium carrots, cut lengthwise and cut in half

4 large Tomatoes, sliced thick

Dressing:

6 tbsp. extra virgin olive oil

Sea salt, to taste

3 tbsp. Balsamic vinegar

Directions:

Dijon mustard Combine all of the dressing ingredients thoroughly. Preheat your grill to low heat and grease the grates. Layer the vegetable grill for 12 minutes per side until tender, flipping once. Brush with the marinade/ dressing ingredients.

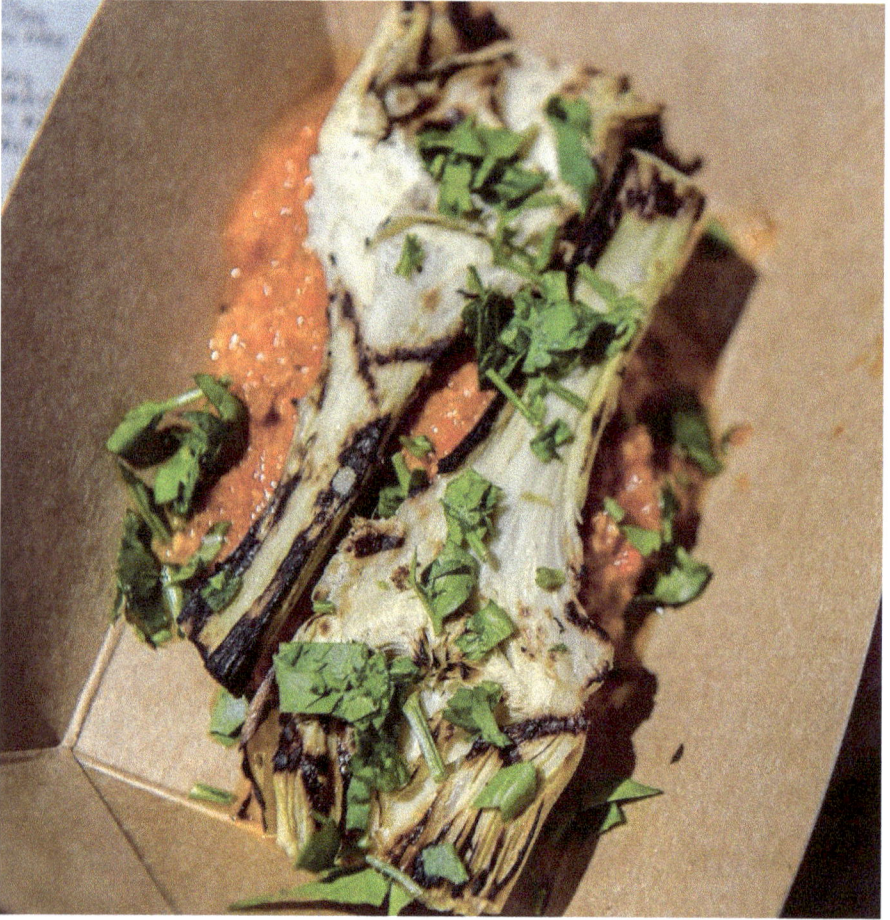

# Grilled Winter Squash and Beets

Ingredients

5 pcs. Beets

1 winter squash, peeled and sliced lengthwise

10 pcs. Brussel Sprouts

1 large red onion, cut into

1/2 inch thick rounds

1/3 cup Italian parsley or basil, finely chopped

Dressing:

6 tbsp. extra virgin olive oil

Sea salt, to taste

3 tbsp. apple cider vinegar

1 tbsp. honey

Directions:

Egg-free mayonnaise Combine all of the dressing ingredients thoroughly. Preheat your grill to low heat and grease the grates. Layer the vegetable grill for 12 minutes per side until tender, flipping once. Brush with the marinade/ dressing ingredients

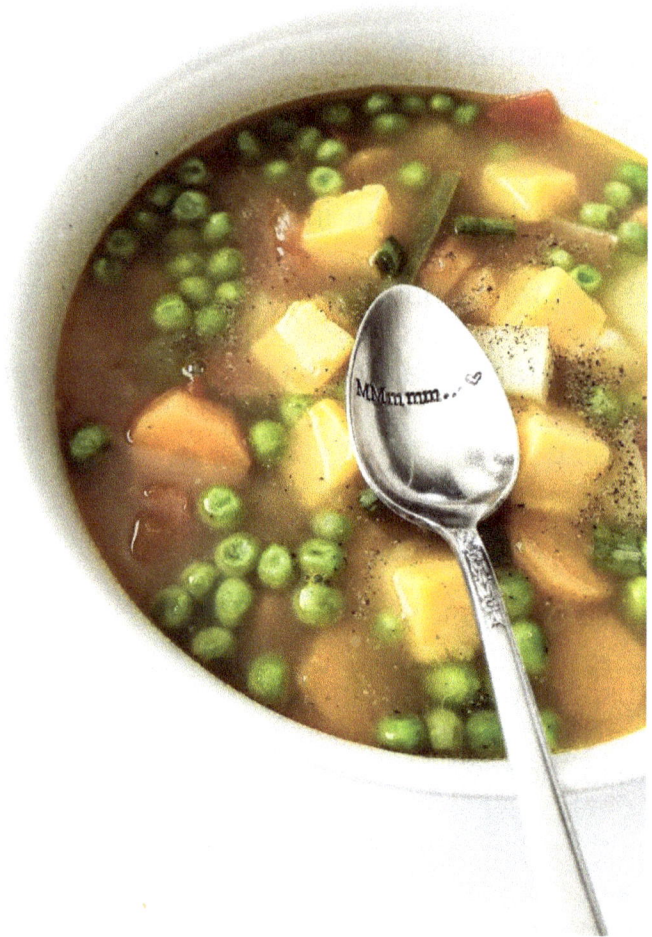

## Grilled Cabbage and Mustard Greens

Ingredients

1 medium Cabbage sliced

1 bunch of mustard greens

1/3 cup Italian parsley or basil, finely chopped

Dressing:

6 tbsp. extra virgin olive oil

Sea salt, to taste

3 tbsp. Balsamic vinegar

Directions:

Combine all of the dressing ingredients thoroughly. Preheat your grill to low heat and grease the grates. Layer the vegetable grill for 12 minutes per side until tender, flipping once. Brush with the marinade/ dressing ingredients

## Grilled Okra and Red Onions

Ingredients

10 pcs. Okra

1 large red onion, cut into

1/2 inch thick rounds

1/3 cup Italian parsley or basil, finely chopped

Dressing:

6 tbsp. olive oil

1 tsp. garlic powder

1 tsp. onion powder

Sea salt, to taste

3 tbsp. white wine vinegar

Directions:

English mustard Combine all of the dressing ingredients thoroughly. Preheat your grill to low heat and grease the grates. Layer the vegetable grill for 12 minutes per side until tender, flipping once. Brush with the marinade/ dressing ingredients

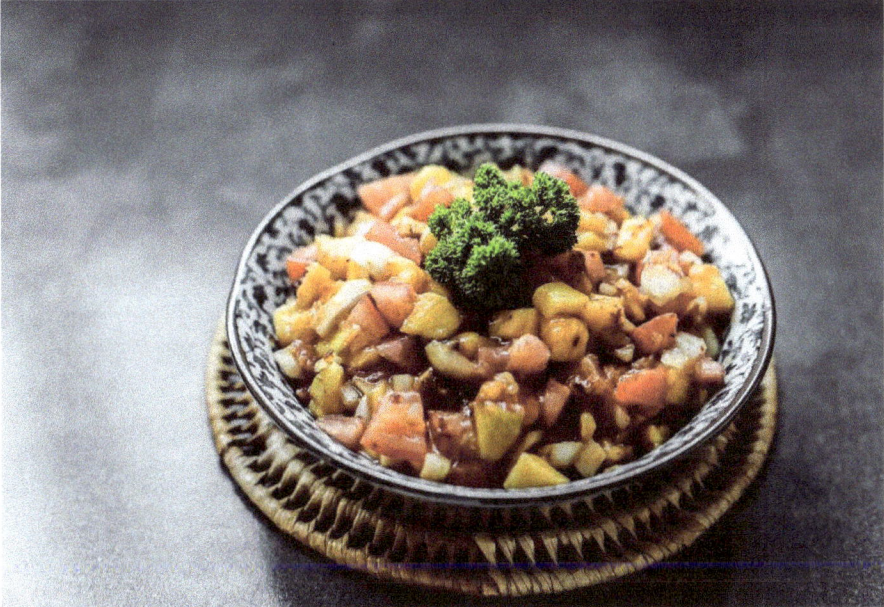

**Sweets**

**Chocolate-chip cookie ice-cream sandwiches**
Prep:20 mins Cook:20 mins  Plus overnight chilling Easy
Makes 12 sandwiches or 24 cookies

Ingredients

280g brown sugar

225g sugar

250g butter

2 large eggs

1 tbsp vanilla extract

450g plain flour

2 tsp baking powder

300g milk chocolate

vanilla ice cream

Directions:

To make the cookies, tip the sugars and butter into a large bowl. Get a grown-up to help you use an electric hand mixer to blend them until the mixture looks smooth and creamy, and a little paler in colour.

Carefully break in the eggs, one at a time, mixing well between each egg and pausing to scrape down the sides with a spatula. Mix in the vanilla.

Sift in the flour and baking powder, then mix well with a wooden spoon.Stir through the chocolate chunks. Use your hands to squeeze the dough together in 1 big lump, split into 2 even pieces. Put each piece on a sheet of cling film.

Roll each piece of dough in the cling film to form thick sausage shapes and then seal the ends. Put them in the fridge and chill for at least 3 hrs or overnight – can be frozen at this point.

Heat oven to 180C/160C fan/ gas 4. Take the dough rolls out of the fridge, unwrap and use a small knife to slice each one into 12 pieces, so you have 24 in total.

Place the slices on a baking tray lined with baking parchment. Put this in the oven to bake for 20 mins or until the cookies are golden brown on the edges, but still pale in the centre.

Allow to cool slightly before lifting them onto a wire rack to cool completely. Sandwich the cookies together with ice cream and dig in!

## Keto Granola Bars

Easy chewy no-bake hemp seeds bars 100% Nut-Free, Grain-Free, and Vegan with only 4.2 grams of net carbs and 9 grams of protein per bar.

Prep Time: 25 mins Total Time: 25 mins 10 granola bars

Ingredients

Dry ingredients

1/2 cup Sunflower seed butter

3 tablespoons Coconut oil

1/4 cup Sugar-free flavored maple syrup

1 teaspoon Vanilla extract

1 cup hemp hearts - raw, shelled also known as hemp seeds

1 tablespoon Chia seeds

1/3 cup Pumpkin seeds

1/4 cup Sunflower seeds

1/3 cup Coconut chips

1/2 teaspoon Cinnamon

2 tablespoons Erythritol - or /3 stevia drops (optional, to adjust sweetness)


Chocolate drizzle

1/4 cup Sugar-free Chocolate Chips 1 teaspoon Coconut oil

## Instructions

Line a 9-inch x 5-inch loaf pan with parchment paper. Set aside.

In a medium mixing bowl, add all the dry ingredients, the order doesn't matter. Stir, set aside.

In another mixing bowl, add sunflower seed butter, melted coconut oil, sugar-free syrup, and vanilla.

Microwave 30 seconds, stir, microwave 30 seconds again if your sunflower seed butter is too hard to combine. You must obtain a thick brownish paste. If you don't have a microwave, bring on a stove in a small saucepan, stirring often until the ingredients are combined.

Pour the seed butter mixture onto the dry ingredients and combine with a spoon until the mixture covers all the dry ingredients evenly.

Transfer the mixture into the prepared loaf pan, press with a spatula firmly to compact the granola bar mixture as much as you can.

Freeze 20 minutes to set.

## Chocolate drizzle

Meanwhile, melt the sugar-free chocolate chips and coconut oil in a small bowl. You can microwave by 30 seconds burst, or use a saucepan under medium heat.

Bring the bar out of the freezer. Lift the parchment paper to pull out the bar from the loaf pan and place it on a plate or chopping board.

Drizzle the melted chocolate on top of the bar and bring the bar back to the freezer for 2 minutes to set the chocolate.

Cut into 10 bars, I recommend you warm the knife blade under a flame or hot water (dry the blade to avoid water to be added to the bar).

Storage and freezing

Store the bars in the fridge in an airtight container for up to 3 weeks or wrap individually into plastic wrap and freeze up to 3 months.

These bars must be kept in the fridge as they soften after 20 minutes out of the fridge.

Nutrition Info

Calories 285 Calories from Fat 224 Fat 24.9g38% Carbohydrates 13.5g Fiber 9.2g38% Protein 9.2g

# Keto Strawberry Pop Tarts

A buttery flaky pastry filled with sugar-free chia seed jam
Prep Time: 15 mins

Cook Time: 20 mins Total Time: 35 mins 8 pop tarts

Ingredients

Keto pastry doughFilling

2 1/4 cup Almond Flour, fine, blanched (250g)

1/2 cup Coconut Flour fresh, no lump, packed, leveled up (60g)

1/4 cup Erythritol - erythritol (swerve) or Monk fruit (Lakanto)

2 1/2 teaspoon Xanthan gum - don't skip!

1/3 cup + 1 tbsp Unsweetened Almond Milk

3.5 oz Melted Unsalted Butter (100g) or dairy-free vegan butter 1/2 tablespoon Apple cider vinegar


To decorate

6 tablespoons Sugar free chia seed jam

6 tablespons Cream Cheese or vegan coconut yoghurt

1/4 cup Sugar-free powdered sweetener

1/2-1 tablespoon Unsweetened Almond Milk adjust to taste


Instructions

Before you start, make sure you measure all the ingredients precisely either in grams/oz or cups. If you use cups firmly pack flours in the cup and level up.

Preheat oven to 180C (350F). Line a baking tray with parchment paper. Set aside.

In a large mixing bowl, whisk all the dry ingredients together : almond flour, coconut flour, sugar-free crystal sweetener and xanthan gum.

Add in unsweetened almond milk, melted butter, and apple cider vinegar.

Combine with a spoon at first then knead the dough with your hands until you are able to shape a ball.

Wrap the pastry dough ball into a piece of parchment paper or cling film wrap.

Freeze 10 minutes.

Remove the dough from the freezer and divide the dough ball in half. Roll each half between two pieces of parchment paper into a 1/4 inches thick rectangles about 1.5 x 2.3 inches ( 4cm x 6 cm). You will get around 16 small rectangles in total, 8 from each half dough balls. For larger tarts, double size of each rectangles and make only 6 pop tarts (net carb will consequently double up too)

Transfer rectangles of dough onto the prepared baking tray, leaving 1 thumb space between each rectangle. The dough won't expand while baking but the jam may run out the pastry so it's better to leave some space between each pop tart.

Spread 1/2 tablespoon of cream cheese (or vegan coconut yoghurt) in the center of each rectangle of dough leaving 1/2 inch (1 cm) border around the edges. Layer 1/2 tablespoon of chia seed jam on each rectangle over the cream cheese and add few slices of fresh strawberries (optional) . Make sure you don't cover the borders of the rectangle with the filling or you won't be able to close the tart. Use less filling if needed (this can happen if you roll your dough thicker and didn't manage to cut out enough rectangles)

Lay the other rectangles over the filling and seal the edges by pressing with your fingertips. If desired, cut the top dough with a knife to form gills - optional.

Brush the top of each pop tarts with beaten eggs or unsweetened almond milk if vegan.

Bake for 25 minutes in the center rack of your until the crust is golden brown. You can add a piece of foil on top of the pop tarts if the crust brown to dark/too fast and bring the tray to a level lower in the oven.

Meanwhile, in a small bowl combine sugar-free powdered sweetener with almond milk. Add more almond milk to make the glazing more liquid or add more powdered sweetener to thicken.

Cool down the pop tarts on a rack for 2 hours. Drizzle the glazing onto the cold pop tarts

Store in an airtight container in the fridge for up to 3 days or freeze individually and defrost the day before at room temperature.

Nutrition Info

Calories 307 Calories from Fat 151 Fat 16.8g Carbohydrates 11g Fiber 4.4g18% Sugar 2.6g3% Protein 6.3g

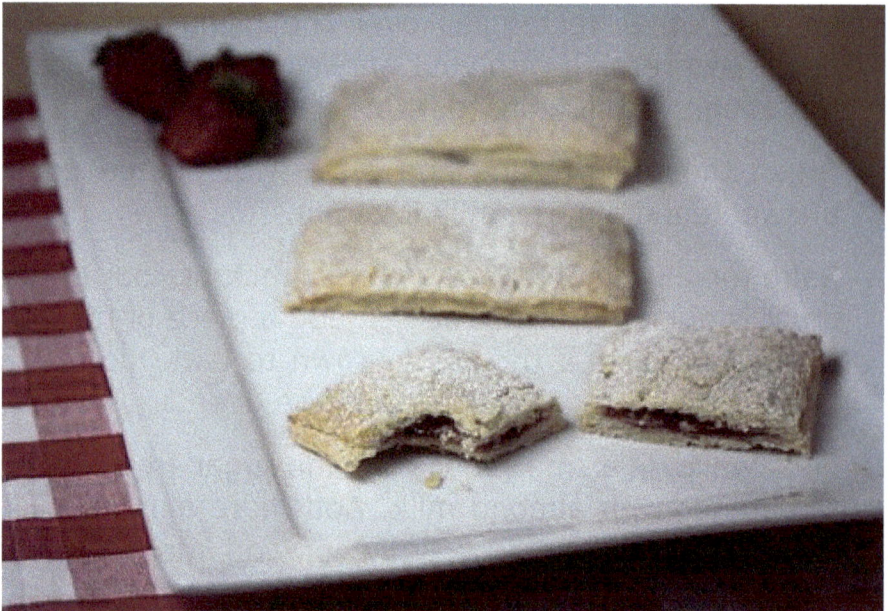

# Crispy chocolate fridge cake

Prep:20 mins Cook:5 mins Plus chilling Easy Makes 16-20 chunks

Ingredients

300g dark chocolate

100g butter 140g golden syrup 2 tsp vanilla extract

220g biscuit

120g sultana 85g Rice Krispies

140g mini eggs

50g white chocolate


Directions:

Line a 20 x 30cm tin with baking parchment. Melt the chocolate, butter and golden syrup in a bowl set over a pan of simmering water, stirring occasionally, until smooth and glossy. Add the vanilla, biscuits, sultanas and Rice Krispies, and mix well until everything is coated.

Tip the mixture into the tin, then flatten it down with the back of a spoon. Press in some mini eggs, if using, and put in the fridge until set. When hard, drizzle all over with the melted white chocolate and set again before cutting into chunks.

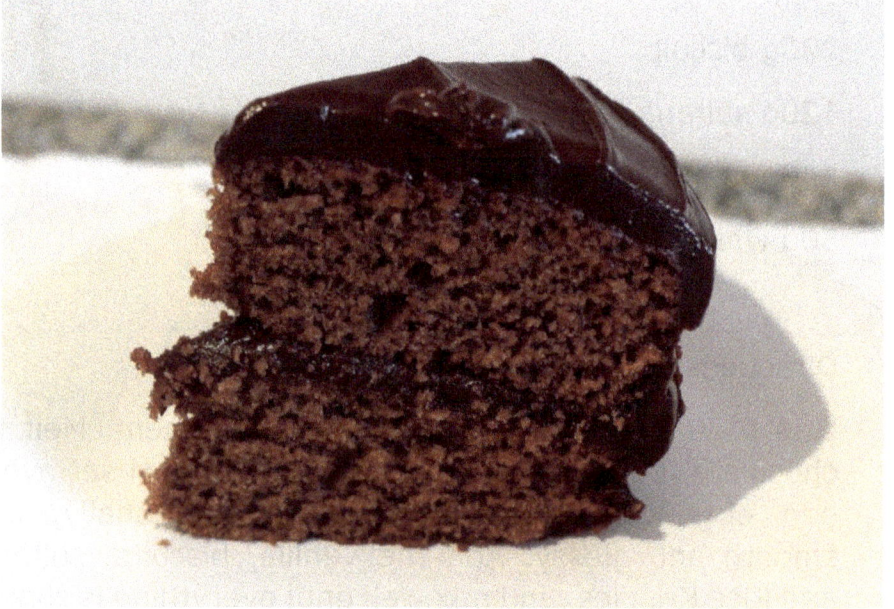

## Oat Applesauce Muffins

Prep time: 15 min Cooking Time: 30 min serve: 2

Ingredients

¼ cup rolled oats ¼ cup buttermilk

¼ cup all-purpose flour ¼ teaspoon baking powder

¼ teaspoon baking soda 1/4 tablespoon honey

½ tablespoon applesauce 1 egg 1 cup water

Instructions

In a large bowl, stir together all-purpose flour, baking powder, baking soda and honey. Stir in oats and buttermilk mixture, applesauce and egg; mix well. Pour batter into prepared muffin cups.

Pour 1 cup water into the Instant Pot. Place the trivet inside. Place the muffin cups on the rack or pan.

Secure the lid and set the Pressure Release valve to Sealing. Press the Pressure Cook or Manual button and set the cook time to 20 minutes.

When the Instant Pot beeps, allow the pressure to release naturally for 10 minutes, then carefully switch the Pressure Release valve to Venting. When fully released, open the lid. Carefully remove the muffins.

Nutrition Facts

Calories 150, Total Fat 3.3g, Saturated Fat 1g, Cholesterol 83mg, Sodium 223mg, Total Carbohydrate

## Marshmallows dipped in chocolate

Prep: 10 mins Cook:5 mins Plus setting time easy Makes 26 approx

Ingredients

50g white chocolate

50g milk chocolate

selection of cake sprinkles

1 bag marshmallows (about 200g)

1 pack lollipop sticks


Directions:

Heat the chocolate in separate bowls over simmering water or on a low setting in the microwave. Allow to cool a little.

Put your chosen sprinkles on separate plates. Push a cake pop or lolly stick into a marshmallow about half way in. Dip into the white or milk chocolate, allow the excess to drip off then dip into the sprinkles of your choice. Put into a tall glass to set. Repeat with each marshmallow.

# Christmas pudding Rice Krispie cakes

Prep: 30 hrs Cook:5 mins plus chilling Easy Makes 10 - 12

Ingredients

50g rice pops (we used Rice Krispies)

30g raisin, chopped 50g butter

100g milk chocolate, broken into pieces

2 tbsp crunchy peanut butter

30g mini marshmallow

80g white chocolate ready-made icing holly leaves


Directions:

Put the rice pops and raisins into a bowl. Put the butter, milk chocolate, peanut butter and marshmallows into a small saucepan. Place on a medium to low heat and stir until the chocolate and butter have melted but the marshmallows are just beginning to melt.

Pour onto the rice pops and stir until well coated. Line an egg cup with cling film. Press about a tablespoon of the mixture into the egg cup. Press firmly and then remove, peel off the cling film and place the pudding into a cake case, flat-side down. Repeat with the remaining mixture. Chill until firm.

Melt the white chocolate in the microwave or bowl over a saucepan of barely simmering water. Spoon a little chocolate over the top of each pudding. Top with icing holly leaves.

## Yummy chocolate log

Prep:30 mins Cook:10 mins More effort Serves 8

Ingredients

For the cake

3 eggs

85g golden caster sugar

85g plain flour (minus 2 tbsp)

2 tbsp cocoa powder

½ tsp baking powder

For the filling & icing • 50g butter, plus extra for the tin

140g dark chocolate, broken into squares

1 tbsp golden syrup

284ml pot double cream

200g icing sugar, sifted

2-3 extra strong mints, crushed (optional)

icing sugar and holly sprigs to decorate - ensure you remove the berries before serving


Directions:

Heat the oven to 200C/180C fan/gas 6. Butter and line a 23 x 32cm Swiss roll tin with baking parchment. Beat the eggs and golden caster sugar together with an electric whisk for about 8 mins until thick and creamy. Mix the flour, cocoa powder and baking powder, then sift onto the egg mixture. Fold in very carefully, then pour into the tin. Tip the tin from side to side to spread the mixture into the corners. Bake for 10 mins.

Lay a sheet of baking parchment on a work surface. When the cake is ready, tip it onto the parchment, peel off the lining paper, then roll the cake up from its longest edge with the paper inside. Leave to cool.

To make the icing, melt the butter and dark chocolate together in a bowl over a pan of hot water. Take from the heat and stir in the golden syrup and 5 tbsp double cream. Beat in the icing sugar until smooth.

Whisk the remaining double cream until it holds its shape. Unravel the cake, spread the cream over the top, scatter over the crushed extra strong mints, if using, then carefully roll up again into a log.

Cut a thick diagonal slice from one end of the log. Lift the log on to a plate, then arrange the slice on the side with the diagonal cut against the cake to make a branch. Spread the icing over the log and branch (don't cover the ends), then use a fork to mark the icing to give tree bark effect. Scatter with unsifted icing sugar to resemble snow, and decorate with holly.

## Easy Easter nests

Prep: 25 mins Cook:8 mins Plus chilling easy Makes 12
Ingredients

200g milk chocolate, broken into pieces

85g shredded wheat, crushed

2 x 100g bags mini chocolate eggs

cupcake cases


Directions:

Melt the chocolate in a small bowl placed over a pan of barely simmering water. Pour the chocolate over the shredded wheat and stir well to combine.

Spoon the chocolate wheat into 12 cupcake cases and press the back of a teaspoon in the centre to create a nest shape. Place 3 mini chocolate eggs on top of each nest. Chill the nests in the fridge for 2 hrs until set.

## Choco-dipped tangerines

Prep: 10 mins Easy Serves 1

Ingredients

1 tangerine, peeled and segmented

10g dark chocolate, melted

Directions:

Dip half of each tangerine segment in the melted chocolate, then put on a baking sheet lined with parchment. Keep in the fridge for 1 hr to set completely, or overnight if you prefer.

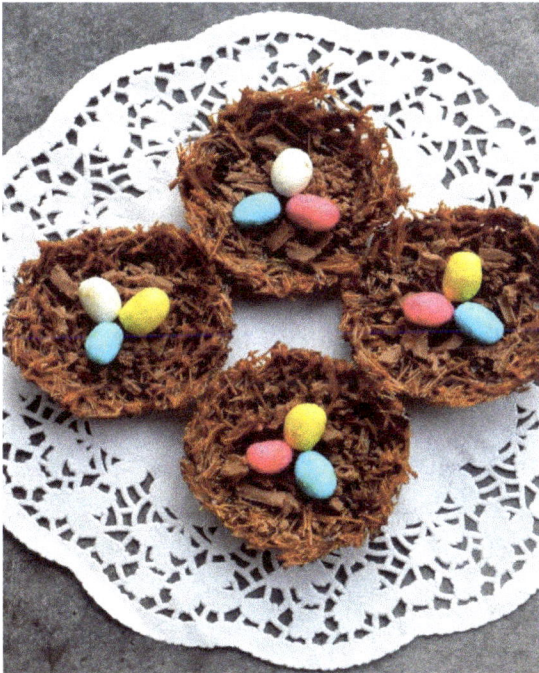

# Chocolate crunch bars

Cook: 5 mins Prep: 20 mins plus chilling Easy Cuts into 12

Ingredients

100g butter, roughly chopped

300g dark chocolate (such as Bournville), broken into squares

3 tbsp golden syrup

140g rich tea biscuit, roughly crushed

12 pink marshmallows, quartered (use scissors)

2 x 55g bars Turkish delight

Directions:

Gently melt the butter, chocolate and syrup in a pan over a low heat, stirring frequently until smooth, then cool for about 10 mins.

Stir the biscuits and sweets into the pan until well mixed, then pour into a 17cm square tin lined with foil and spread the mixture to level it roughly. Chill until stiff, then cut into fingers.

www.ingramcontent.com/pod-product-compliance
Lightning Source LLC
Chambersburg PA
CBHW050756030426
42336CB00012B/1850